FIRST RESPONDER

As seen through my eyes

Based on a true story

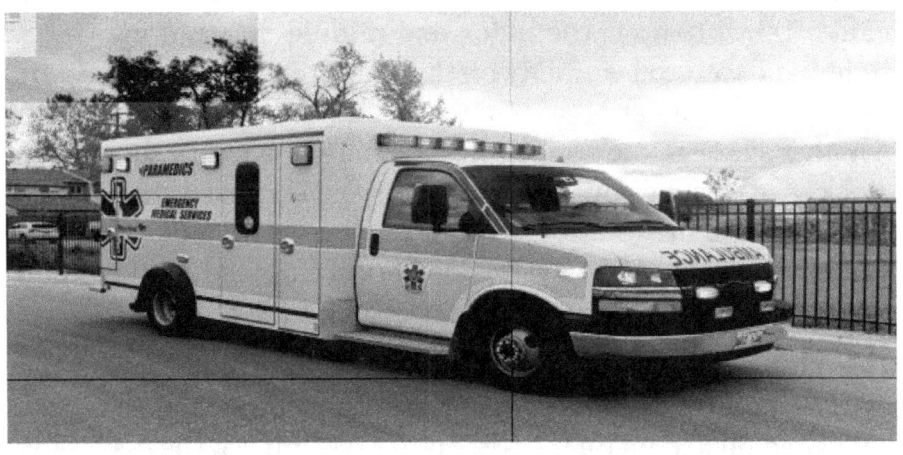

Written by Timothy Guy

Assisted by Mary Louise

CHAPTER ONE

EMT Brad, racing to the hospital, quickly radios dispatch for assistance. His partner Tim is in the back of the ambulance with a pregnant woman whose baby is "crowning"; however, something is wrong! Tim determines there is not enough time to wait for dispatch to contact the hospital.

In training we were briefed on such a situation and thank God I paid attention. I put the index and middle finger of my gloved right hand into the women's birth canal and I could feel the cord. Now comes the hard part, I must decide to move the cord, but which way? I can't see anything, just a slight touch. I sensed that clockwise was the correct choice, so I gently moved the cord and out came the baby, whoosh! Lucky I was an infielder with soft hands; mother and baby were both fine. I clamped off the umbilical cord just as we arrived at the hospital.

Thinking back, it was the summer of '72 when we received that call from the dispatcher. So much can happen in only 15 minutes. EMT Brad picked up on the first ring, EMS Unit #5, the dispatcher said, "respond to four nine two one W. Monroe, woman in labor, again that is 4921 W. Monroe, woman in labor". Brad runs out to the ambulance, jumps in the driver's seat, looks to his partner Tim in the jump seat for the best route and away we drive, two First Responders helping in any way we can. Little did I know that this would be the first of many such experiences in the city of Detroit over my next six, and one-half years as a First Responder.

I was waiting for Brad in the loading area after we dropped off the lady and baby, just sitting in the jump seat (passenger) of the ambulance chuckling over a story my mother used to tell about my birth. My father worked for a trucking company at the time and when my mom finally got hold of him at one of his stops and said she needed to go to the hospital, he responded, just hold your legs together, I have one more stop. Little did I know as the second son about hand me downs, etc. Remember this is the early 50's, no cell phones. By the time he arrived it was too late to go to her regular hospital in Detroit, so the closest hospital was in Grosse Point, a very wealthy neighborhood compared to Detroit City. I am the only member of my 4 brothers not born in Detroit, but up-scale Grosse Point, and lived there for a total of 3 days.

By the 60's my father was a Firefighter, also a First Responder. Back then, the Firefighters responded to all medical emergencies. The creation of the Emergency Medical Service, EMS, created quite a bit of controversy with Firefighters. Many were relieved not to be responding to medical emergencies. However, not everyone felt that way and many of the older men felt we were not only replacing them, but also imposing on their daily activities in the firehouse. The average age of the EMT's was considerably younger the firefighters, and back in the early 70's experience was everything and youth was not respected.

My parents were not financially able to send 5 sons to college, so they decided to send us to a Catholic Elementary school and an all-boys high school. My older brother and I graduated from this highly rated college preparatory school. The day after I graduated, I applied for a job as an orderly at St. Johns Hospital on the east side, bordering Harper Woods, Detroit and Grosse Point. The lady in charge of the interview was an African American, quite unusual in 1970. I was only 17, having graduated a year early, and was not doing very well in the interview when she noticed I graduated from De La Salle and the tone of the interview completely changed. I got the job and I was incredibly surprised.

About 18 months passed by and my father took me to apply for the EMS, they were taking 600 applicants to whittle down to just over 60. I was at Wayne State University taking basic liberal arts requirements, very boring, and some medical pre-requisite courses. I was offered an opportunity to test for the EMT position, along with 600 other folks. The test was not extremely hard, having 18 months of Emergency Room on the job experience coupled with my Anatomy & Physiology and other medical courses I had just completed at Wayne State. Then came the physical requirements. Lucky for me I was in excellent shape. Not the biggest guy, however; I was lean, quick and strong for my size, about 5'10" and 165.

I found out later that I came in second in the physical and first in the exam, wow! Obviously, I was offered the job and promoted to EMT Technician and assigned an EMT Trainee. I was not even 20 years old yet and most of the people hired were corpsman from the military in their late 20's and early 30's. Many of them were not pleased to be a trainee and this young kid a Technician. I chose to ignore their attitude and tried to work together. The EMT in the jump seat did most of the patient triage and emergency treatment and the partner drove the ambulance and provided any additional assistance. On a couple occasions I was forced to take a stand when unnecessarily questioned by the older fellas. I simply told them we took the same exam and had the same physical test. I did considerably better and that was the end of it. Growing up in Detroit you learned to have a loud bark, even without much of a bite, and most people respected you standing up for yourself.

The opportunity I had at the hospital was extremely exciting; however, at the Fire Department as a First Responder it was considerably more exciting as well as better compensation. I bought a new Gremlin X. You can laugh now; I liked the car. Unfortunately, while driving to work one evening, working the 11pm to 7:30 am, I was driving in the middle lane of the freeway in my EMS uniform when I saw a car coming over the guard rail and aiming for me. Holly shit! I dove onto the floor of the passenger side, no seat belts then, and prayed. When the vehicle stopped spinning, I placed my fingers on the passenger door's window, slowly raising up to peak out the window at the oncoming traffic. My little Gremlin X was sitting sideways in the middle of the freeway and several vehicles were bearing down on me; luckily, they all stopped in time.

The lady driving the huge Pontiac Catalina was drunk; her driver's side front bumper hit just behind the driver's door of my vehicle and as I said, knocked me spinning. The EMS Unit showed up at the wreck. It was from my station, and I was scheduled as one of their replacements. I suffered a large bruise to my abdomen when I dove onto the floor. I jammed myself into the stick shift and was very, very, lucky. Both the drunken lady, and I were bruised and shaken up without any major injuries, which was quite unusual. We were lucky that when she hit me, I was driving in the middle lane without any surrounding traffic; I always try to drive in between the groups of cars for safety. Unfortunately, I was not allowed to work my shift. I was ready to go, but they were smarter and knew in about 3-4 hours I would be hurting all over and they were correct.

A few weeks later I had a new partner named Casey, a tall good looking sharp Black man; it was a normal rotation and all the EMTs rotated partners. We hit it off well and I am proud to say that we had each other's back. He was a lot stronger and a real gentleman. We had several incidents including the call for a recent veteran who came home from Vietnam and was wilting away in the bed. The call was for a sick man, and as always, we responded. Most of the homes that we entered were in sad to extremely sad condition, but not this home. On the outside the owner had to look "not too good" or they become a target for thieves and who knows what. I entered one of the nicest, cleanest homes I had ever been in. A couple in their 50's took us to the frail son. I was on jump seat, so I asked the parents, both very sharp and smart people what was going on. They could not get their son to go for any help. He refused, and they had tried ambulances, police and EMS before, but he refused to go. My partner was a Vietnam vet and this young man was also. For a lack of the proper term, he was Shell Shocked. His eyes looked at me with such despair; we had to help, somehow. All, of a sudden there were 2 Blue Doberman Pinchers loose in the house. The father told them to sit and instantly they both stopped the attack on the white stranger. The dogs were protecting the son; they knew he was sick. Eventually, we convinced the son to let us help him. Casey was cool and even petted the dogs; I only saw their big white teeth. I have always been a dog lover and between Casey as a fellow black vet and this young man's parents, we got him to agree to get help by convincing him that if one of the dogs was in his condition, he would take it to the veterinarian. A few months later the mother came by the firehouse telling us how her son had recovered, and she even brought us a homemade pie. I did not cry then, but I am now.

The EMS had a lot of rules. The powers in charge of the EMS decided that if a pregnant women's contractions were 2 minutes apart or less it was an emergency and the EMS would respond. So many waited too long because they were alone and poor, and we delivered several babies.

We responded to one woman in labor and got her to the hospital elevator where she delivered between floors. A couple days later we just happen to be dropping off a patient when she was being wheelchaired out. Casey had delivered her baby and went over to see her. Her face was beaming, and he asked her what she named him. She said she named him Otis, why it just came to me! I was fighting off a chuckle which she did not see, but Casey did. After she left, he told me I was prejudiced, and Otis was a good name. Remember he was 6 inches taller than me and at least 40 pounds of muscle. I walked him over to the elevator. When he delivered the baby he was in the doorway and I was facing the door, I turned him around and picked him up by the lapels of his jacket in the doorway of the elevator and asked him to tell me what he saw, "Oh shit Tim" he said. There in bold capital letters was OTIS Elevator Company. To this day every time I get in an elevator, I look above the doorway and most of the time it is the OTIS Elevator Company. You have got to love life!

When the lady delivered the baby in the elevator her posterior water broke and splashed on Casey's winter uniform coat. He was always well dressed and took the coat to the cleaners several times. Unfortunately, it never lost the scent because everywhere he wore that coat dogs would appear and follow him. After a while, as the firefighters would tease him about it so much, he burned the coat behind the firehouse one day.

After a couple years all the EMS units were put on 12-hour shifts, Sunday, Monday Tuesday or Thursday, Friday, Saturday, starting at 7am and 7 pm with a rotating Wednesday. The busier EMS Units were in the more violent areas and usually responded to 20-25 calls on a 12-hour shift, especially on the Friday and Saturday 7 pm to 7 am shift.

One Saturday on a hot and very humid night shift we responded to a stabbing call for another unit already on a call. The response time was over 5 minutes from our area to theirs, so the police were already there. I was on jump seat and entered an incredibly old rundown property and I was behind 4-5 police officers. All, of a sudden, a very, large black man was at the top of the stairs with a bloody hatchet coming at all of us at the foot of the stairs. The first officer in the front shot the man with his 38 police issue pistol; it did not even slow him down. He was extremely drunk, drugged or both. As he started back down waving the hatchet at us, a black police officer pushed the officer that had fired out of the way and shot the attacker 3 times in the chest with his "Dirty Harry" 45. The first shot stopped the attacker in his tracks, the second lifted him up in the air and the third bullet forced him back up against the wall. It is hard to understand the power and destruction of weapons until you "actually" witness it firsthand.

Unfortunately, all the EMTs witnessed so much trauma and violence it made us appear that sometimes we did not care, but the truth is that we had to do our jobs and provide on-site instant care. I remember when I was an orderly in the Emergency Room standing by a young boy that had just passed away, feeling sad because we had helped him several times before. We did not realize that a patient in the next room was having a heart attack and while we wasted time grieving, it almost cost that man his life. It was a painful lesson to learn!

One of the more common calls was for a stroke or heart attack. There were several occasions where my partner and I did Cardio-Pulmonary Resuscitation, (CPR), with positive results. I remember reviving a man in the basement of his home on the East side, by Heilman Park where I learned to ice skate, and when we got him outside in his driveway he had another cardiac arrest and we administered CPR again until the dispatcher could send a second unit. We continued in the ambulance after the second unit arrived, one EMT working the chest and the other attempting to fill the lungs with air and, of course, one driving to the hospital. When we left the hospital, he was awake and out of danger for the moment, but like so many seniors we responded to at that time, he was very overweight and a cigarette smoker.

The Firefighters and the Police were frequently together, at one firehouse the police would chip in and eat a meal with the fireman. I got to know several officers quite well to the point we would party together off duty. One of the worst calls we responded to was, a "police officer down", shot by a criminal while in the process of their duty. On one occasion we responded to an officer down I was driving. After we administered first aid and loaded him into the ambulance, we started to the hospital. The police had the red lights all blocked for me to proceed at top speed. At one of the intersections the police had blocked the red light, it was 3 lanes total and 2 semitrucks with trailer pulled over on each side, so I shot the gap scared it was too tight. As I exited between the 2 trucks I looked to the passenger outside mirror and it was flat against the side of the ambulance. I looked at the drivers outside mirror, and it was flat against the ambulance, another holy shit!

The police had the freeway blocked off, so I had no interference to the hospital. Luckily, the officer lived and came to the firehouse to thank us personally after he recovered, another great feeling when you knew you made a difference.

About a year later I was at a bachelor party on the west side for an EMT and we did the normal things that young men do at their last party as free men. Drinking, smoking, and all the other dumb things men do. After several hours of partying I left to drive home with an open beer. I was maybe 5 minutes on the road, and I got pulled over by the Detroit Police, still with the open beer. Holy shit! I exited the vehicle and there was a white and a black police officer. The white officer told me to assume the position to be handcuffed for drinking and driving. I got my Firefighter badge out when I got my driver's license out and the black officer looked at my badge and back at me a couple times. He said to me are you the First Responder that responded to the shot officer? Of course, I said yes. He looked at me and said laughing, "dump out the beer, put out the smoke and drive safely home"; it was 3 am. I was a bit confused, so he proceeded to tell me it was his partner that was shot that night and he would have recognized me sooner except he said "all you white EMTs look the same". We both laughed, wow!

CHAPTER TWO

I think what initially led me to wanting to become an Emergency Medical Technician was from my job working at a hospital while in high school. The summer before my 16th birthday I got a job working in the kitchen at St. John's Hospital. At first, I pushed the food carts containing patient meals to all floors, both East and West wings. After lunch and dinner, I collected all the trays and pushed all the food carts individually back to the area in the kitchen for cleaning the dishes. Every night 3-4 of us would run the conveyor belt system and rinse, stack, wash and then set up for the next meal.

I did not like going into the patients' rooms because of all the sick people. They had tubes attached and I thought they always had a terrible smell. Remember I was only 15 years old. After a couple months one of the ladies working in the kitchen was out for maternity leave and I volunteered for her work. The job was cutting the vegetables every day for the patients' meals as well as the cafeteria that fed all the employees and family of the patients. I liked this far better than seeing all the sick people in the hospital.

As time went by, I noticed that there are a lot of women working in this hospital compared to the number of men. I also started to notice, after I turned 16, that there were many very, attractive young ladies, some nurses, nurse's aides, clerical workers and even the candy stripers.

At the end of the summer I went back to school and worked part time at the hospital, 4 hours in the evening and one or two full shifts on the weekend. I graduated from De La Salle the summer of 1970 and as I related earlier, I took the opportunity at the hospital to work as an orderly in the emergency room.

I had been in the ER about 18 months when I met Dianne in the elevator under the most unusual circumstances. The morgue was in the basement, down the hall from the Medical Records Department where she worked. When a patient dies in the ER their body is taken down to the morgue in the elevator previously mentioned. One day I was transporting a dead body to the morgue and Dianne and I were in the elevator alone with the corpse. Suddenly, the body sat up! She was scared to death. Rigor-mortis I told her later. Well she was so shocked that she jumped into my arms; was I surprised! Talk about an unusual introduction. The elevator opened, she smiled at me and walked to the Medical Records department where she worked. Just before she opened the door she glanced back and caught me "checking her out" in her pink sweater and black skirt.

I was determined to get to know her better and for 2 weeks I tried to "bump" into her; however, it did not happen. Finally, one day we were in the "elevator" alone, so I started a conversation and she was very friendly. We "bumped" into each other several more times before I got up the courage to ask her out. She accepted, and we dated for almost 3 years.

Shortly after we started going out, I accepted the opportunity at the Detroit Fire Department as an Emergency Medical Technician, EMT. A couple years later we were married, but unfortunately, the marriage did not survive, and we got an annulment from the Catholic Church.

"The Detroit Fire department began providing dedicated ambulance treatment and transport services the summer of 1972, with the mission to provide the citizens and visitors of Detroit with compassionate and professional emergency medical care. The city now has over 900 licensed individuals staffing over 60 vehicles and responding to over 120,000 calls for service annually" (copied from the Detroit Fire Department website June

2020). I thought a little factual history would help to show the overwhelming devotion and hard work put forth by the First Responders.

One evening shift I was working at the unit on the far west side at Joy and Southfield with a new partner, Don. He was a very rough character, 2 tours in Vietnam. He had 3 large shepherds named Killer, Maimer and Destroyer. About 2 AM on a Saturday morning we got a call for a "man down" just up the street in the "projects". I was in the jump seat so when we pulled up at the location, he reminded me not to stand in front of the door when I knocked, I rolled my eyes and headed to the door.

To humor Don, I stepped to the side and knocked on the door, the door exploded into splinters due to both barrels of a shotgun being fired! The "man down" had been beaten and robbed, so he crawled to get his gun determined to get them when they came back. The next thing I knew I was standing on the corner of the block; Don never got out of the driver's seat. He smoked the tires to get to where I was standing. The first thing he said was "man I can't believe you cleared that hedge" laughing. I looked back and there was an 8 feet tall hedge. The next thing I noticed was that my right leg was all wet. I did it, it was urine, Don laughed again. After the police arrived, we transported the injured man to the hospital and at the hospital I had several splinters removed from my back, nothing major, I finished my shift. I never stood in front of a door when I knocked ever again; experience is the best teacher.

There are many coincidences in life that we all experience. My unit received a call for an auto accident, injured woman. The accident was in another unit's area and frequently we all would fill in when the other unit is already busy. I again was in the jump seat and when we arrived, I found a young lady with a cut on her face, not too bad, however she was more concerned about her new Camaro. The other driver was drunk and faded over the yellow line into on coming traffic and she did a great job to almost completely avoid him. Unfortunately, when the drunk's vehicle did strike her, she hit her face on the steering wheel. I was not aware as to why I was being so nice to her, but a few months later I would find out when a friend set me up on a blind date.

I was sleeping in one of my partner's basement with their cats and after a month or so a friend of mine, a Detroit Police Officer, set me up a blind date.

I was very hesitant, but he talked me into going. We were to meet these 2 young ladies at a bar called the Purple Grape in Detroit; they had live music and it was very, popular. The two young ladies were attractive, and I was matched up with the blonde and my friend was with the brunette. It did not take long to realize the blonde was not interested in me; she was more interested in my friend, the cop. The brunette lady kept looking over at me several times with a quizzical look on her face. My friend realized that the blonde was more interested in him and asked her to dance; I felt relieved. So, I started to talk to the brunette; of course, her name was also Diane. As we talked, she appeared to get very, excited. Finally, she blurted out "you are the Emergency Medical Technician that responded to my car accident." OMG, this was the young lady with the Camaro. What an unbelievable coincidence that 6 or more months later we met on a blind date, the only one I was ever on. We became good friends and dated for a while, but I had been single just a few months and was scared to get involved in a relationship so soon.

On the next rotation of partners, I was matched up with Bill. He was a Vietnam veteran, a corpsman, who had been promoted several times for his heroism. We made quite a pair; he was about my size with long wavy, curly, red hair in a ponytail. He was married and had 2 children. I really liked Bill, we hit it off well from the beginning. We had several incidents that I remember. One was the case of a young man who appeared to have committed suicide. He lived in an upstairs apartment, renting from an older lady that called 911 because she could not get him to respond. The older lady could not go up the steps but was concerned because he did not respond to her attempts for 2-3 days. We entered the home and went up the stairs to find the renter naked in the bed surrounded by 300-400 pills of every color spilled out on the bed. The young man was dead, although he still had an erection, laying in the pile of pills, very strange. Bill needed to go to the bathroom, so he used the bathroom upstairs while we waited for the police, in the bathroom he found two large shopping bags full of marijuana. After the police arrived, we got another run and left the deceased to the coroner.

In the 1970's the Fire Department was under pressure to hire more females and blacks, so the exam and the physical requirements were made more attainable. I was chosen to have one of the first lady EMTs and was not real, happy about it. I thought I would always get stuck with the most physical work as well as to have to protect her, but could she protect me. The lady assigned as my partner was an African American lady, a Registered Nurse, and possibly the most attractive black lady I ever saw. We became good friends and my fears were all unnecessary. Every run we went on she would ask the men hanging around if they would carry the stretcher or assist us in any way we wanted; they always agreed. Beauty has power! I never had any of the problems that would confront two male, white EMTs because of her. She had a way with men no matter what condition they were in. I was very, lucky to have her as my partner, a very classy, educated lady. It was just the opposite of what I had expected.

The scheduling system had each EMT working three days a week, 12 hours, with the same partner and on the rotating Wednesdays, we had a different partner. One of these partners was Joe, a nice man, with a handlebar mustache, and a bit different. Joe's dad was a professional gambler. He had played tennis against a couple of professionals as well as beating the pro bowlers, both for big money. We would play poker at his house during Monday night football. One Saturday we went to the police auction and bought a poker table. We recovered it with green felt and would have 4-6 guys over at his house for poker.

One evening we responded to a shooting; it was drug and gang related, there were close to 100 bystanders and multiple police-men. The victim had the back of his head blown off all over the white painted wall, very gory. Joe drove back to the firehouse to get his personal camera so he could take pictures, a bit strange if you ask me.

Joe used to go the car auctions and he bought a 1969 Corvette Stingray which I later purchased from him. It was a little beaten-up and had a lot of miles on it and had a 427 with tri-power, 3 car-buretors, and 400 horsepower. I never realized that this car could attract females like it did, young ladies would see the car coming and cross the street to try and hitch a ride. If I met someone and we walked out to the parking lot, they would never walk toward the Vet; it was too cool for me. I fixed up the vehicle to include a new fancy paint job, Hooker headers, Crager mags, etc. The Vet had air conditioning, power windows, tee tops and a great stereo, a babe magnet.

It is the only vehicle I have ever owned that you could just go for a ride without any other plans and still have a good time just driving. I would get a date and bring a bottle of wine and go for a long drive on a sunny day with the t- tops out and enjoy the roar the engine produced through the chrome headers. I always had to be to warn the passenger about getting out of the Vet to be very, careful, not to touch the headers with her leg because they were super-hot, a lesson I learned the hard way. To be completely hon-est, it was also the most expensive vehicle to repair. I had a friend working at the local Chevy dealer in the parts department and I came in for a part that was $6.95 unless it was for the Vet, and it was $27.95 for the exact same part, something to do with the turn signals and emergency lights motor. He took care of me.

CHAPTER 3

Every First Responder sees so much trauma whether it be a vehicle accident, shooting, stabbing, beating, robbery, or a fallen senior, it all adds up in your head. After several years of daily contact with the most gruesome experiences that only soldiers in combat experience, it forces you to either harden or go nuts. To this day I will react to something that brings back sad memories that "you had to be there" to fully grasp; no one understands. My wife says it was over 40 years ago, "let it go", but we, cannot!

The first call I responded to for a dead baby was not crib death; the dead baby was in the dumpster in the alley and then there was the woman that delivered in the toilet who said, "welfare only pays for 5 I already got 7", not easy to ever forget. Twice I responded to same address for the same stepfather stabbed. One time his intestines were exposed and "leaking out", but he refused to press charges against the stepson. One of the weirdest calls was a motorcycle accident at rush hour on a Friday. The motorcycle rider was decapitated, but we could not find the head until a young boy ran up and told us it had rolled down the street. The head was still in the helmet 3 houses away. One of the most uncomfortable experiences was my unit responding to a rape of a young, well developed teenaged black girl. Two male EMTs responded. I was in the jump seat, so I had to get in the back of the ambulance with her and get some information on what happened, as no one else was with her. How do you think she felt, after what she went through, to be stuck in the back of small ambulance with another man, a white man, she must have been terrified! I remember the sadness in this young lady's eyes. I doubt I will ever forget.

Back in the early 70's many vehicles did not have seat belts or people refused to use them if available. The most gruesome vehicle accidents I responded to were involving the passenger seat in a van. Without a seatbelt in an accident the driver's impact was with the steering wheel and the passenger was launched thru the windshield. Before safety glass, they would experience multiple facial and upper body lacerations, quite bloody.

I had a friend with a late 60's van, and I would never sit in the passenger seat when we would drive to Ontario for ice time to practice hockey. I was not particularly good, my mother had given me figure skates years before, but I never had hockey skates until I was 19 and bought them myself. I had little to no skill with the hockey stick other than to be able to "poke check" the puck away from the opposition. I was an extremely fast skater, so I was the fourth line center and my job was to pester the hell out of the puck carrier on the other team; I liked it.

My next-door neighbor was a good hockey player and every year his team would play a game with the Red Wing Oldtimers, ex professionals who were retired. One year they had a player no show so at the last minute, and being right next door, they asked me if I wanted to play. "Hell yes!" was my answer. I did get a little ice time in the game, man were they good, skating circles around us at twice our age. They had several extra rules that made it harder for them, like they had to make 4 consecutive successful passes before a shot; they still beat us 10-1, they were not happy about the one our guys scored. The moment was special, playing in the old Olympia Stadium where the Red Wings would play the next night, cool!

I was at Olympia Stadium a few weeks later when our unit responded as backup when one of the Flying Wallendas had a fall without a net the man was crushed, and he died.

I experienced several less traumatic incidents, such as the time the call came from dispatch over the radio to the home two friends and I were renting. It was quite a shock to hear "guns fired" from the dispatcher. One of my roommates Rick, called in the shooting because the white people on one side and the black people on the other side were shooting at each other with him in the middle. No one was injured although several were jailed, and Rick had one hell of a story to tell. He was, also the first person I ever met that tried to emulate characters from the "Hobbit."

One of the incidents that shows the depravity of humans involved a call for a young boy with something stuck in his ear. It took a few minutes for him to calm down and let the "white man" try to get a hold of whatever was in there with a hemostat, after a few minutes I pulled out a live cock roach. If you saw the filthy condition of the home, it was not too unbelievable.

At one of the EMS Units I pulled an overtime shift; they had a huge, I mean really, huge German Shepherd, King. The lowest form of locals would call in a fake call and after the fireman drove off they would sneak in before the doors closed and rob them, even to the point of taking the steaks off their plates at dinnertime; it was timed perfectly! So, the fireman got King, about 150-175 pounds and with his front paws on my shoulders he was looking down at me. Nobody ever got in after the fireman pulled out again, including me.

My first day there a call came in for the firefighters, not the Emergency Medical Service, so I watched the engine and hook and ladder pull out. Unfortunately, I was outside the doors when the trucks left and when I attempted to enter, King turned into one mean dog. I watched the doors close from outside the firehouse. This neighborhood was extremely dangerous, especially for a white person. I hid in the shadow of the doorway hoping it was a false alarm, and didn't want to have to hide out there very long. Luckily for me, the fireman were back quickly and had a belly laugh seeing me hiding in the doorway. They never let me forget it.

I was in college studying for an Associate of Science degree as an Orthopedic Physician's Assistant while I was working as a First Responder. One of the more unique incidents involved an auto accident where I put a pneumatic splint for a broken leg on a victim shortly before my shift ended. We dropped him off at Detroit General Hospital. I was doing an internship at Detroit General Hospital for my Orthopedic Physician's Assistant program and later that day I was casting the same victim's leg that I had splinted a few hours earlier. The man was under the influence of more than alcohol, not violent at all, just blitzed. After I completed the casting, in my hospital outfit, white coat and all, the man asked me if I had a brother in the fire department, I laughed. I did let him in on the joke and we both laughed, as I was leaving, he yelled out "I guess I got the right man for the job!"

One of the first things we learned was to not let ourselves get in a position to be harmed, including the commute to and from the firehouse. One day I was driving to work in my work car, a 60's Dodge Polara, and 3 men tried to rob me at a stop light. The car behind me pulled up to my back bumper and even though I left several feet between me and the vehicle in front of me, that car started to back up to pin me in. I realized what was happening and rammed the vehicle in front of me accidentally pinning one thief between the cars. He was seriously injured, and I sped off to work, only 5 minutes away.

As I entered the firehouse a call came in from dispatch "man down vehicle involved." You got it, it was the thief, I had broken one of his legs. His friends were gone; I put the pneumatic splint on, and we took him to the hospital. I asked him what happened, he made up some bullshit story, but never recognized me. My partner and I laughed about it all night long, carjacking gone wrong. What a world!

Some of the more frequent calls were for overdoses on heroine, far more then one would expect. The junkies would frequently place their friends in a bathtub full of ice cubes when they would overdose. I saw this multiple times. Back in the 70's the

Emergency Room would inject Narcan, and the victim would recover quickly. On several occasions we responded to the same residence and the same victim had overdosed. On one occasion after being given Narcan, that victim pissed on my partner, Phil, yelling at him "you ruined my high!" A couple weeks later we got a call and the same jerk overdosed. Phil, my partner, was working the jump seat and had this fool in the back of the ambulance on the way to the hospital. As I stated before, we become hardened by the environment and so many gruesome experiences. Well heroin is a respiratory depressant, at least that is my opinion, and so junkies would just "forget to breathe", so we would slap them on the chest to get them to inhale. Phil was hardened to the point that he was reading a textbook on the way to the hospital and every couple of minutes I would hear a loud slap to the junkie's chest to get him to breathe. He was not going to let him die, even if he deserved to, he was hardened, but still compassionate.

Another night we responded to an overdose victim, who was in an iced bathtub; we fished her out and one of the bystanders told us she had been a singer with Diana Ross and the Supremes until they had replaced her a few years earlier. What a sick world.

All the experiences were not negative; some were positive lifelong lessons like the afternoon I entered a house fire to rescue a baby girl. I never went into a fire again. It singed my ears and while crawling on the floor and I rubbed my face raw in a couple of spots. If you ever see a person standing up in a house fire without any protection on television, it is totally misleading. Heat rises, and it will fry your lungs if you stand up in a fire and inhale.

Weekend evenings were always super busy, especially in the worst neighborhoods because of the violence and shootings. On one occasion I had a newly hired EMT as my partner, as he was so new, he drove, and I was in the jump seat. We responded to a shooting. Not knowing what he was doing he drove past the police and stopped in front of the house where they were still shooting. One shot came through the passenger door where I was seated; another hit the radio between our seats. I jumped out of the ambulance and dove behind a large tree as 2 or 3 more shots hit the tree, I was bleeding from the head, but not shot, I hit the tree so hard I cut my own head. Finally, the police appeared and shot the shooter. I looked at my new partner, blood dripping down my face, asked him if he was insane to put us in that position. He was freaked out and did not respond. I guarantee he never pulled up to a shooting before the shots stopped again. Rookies!

The response time for the Emergency Medical Service was considerably faster than the police, usually around 3.5 minutes. We were a bit "Gung-ho" and in some neighborhoods not as busy as the police department. I remember responding to shootings and arriving a couple minutes before the police, so we would sit "around the corner" from the shooting, waiting. One incident that we responded to there were several young kids that ran up to the ambulance to tell us where the shooting was, but we had to wait. We were not allowed to have a weapon, no guns, nothing. A couple minutes later the police got there, and we safely followed them to the location and provided first aid to the victims. We cannot help if we are the victims!

CHAPTER 4

I have a major affection for dogs, you know "man's best friend." I have been blessed with several special bubbas and one of them was a pure breed Newfoundland, 198 pounds of happiness.

"The massive Newfoundland is a strikingly, large working dog of heavy bone and dignified bearing. The sweet-tempered Newfie is a famously good companion and has earned a reputation as a patient and watchful "nanny dog" for kids." (copied from the AKC website)

One Saturday afternoon I was painting the trim and gutters on our home, up the ladder about 30-35 feet (two story home), with Dingy, the name I gave the Newfie, under the ladder working on a bone. I had visited the local butcher and bought a femur bone for him to chew on. So, every few minutes I would look down to check on him. One time he was not there. I started to scan the front yard and saw the neighbor's 5-year old boy walking down the driveway towards the street, as his ball rolled into the street. I noticed there was a parked car in front of the home and just before the boy stepped out beyond the parked car, Dingy, who had walked slowly over 50 feet, very gently bumped him in the chest with his head, causing the boy to sit down and start crying. Almost simultaneously, a truck drove over the ball and it rattled the ball several times underneath until it exploded. That is what would have happened to the boy except for the dog's actions!

The wife was supposed to be watching the boy, but she had gone inside because the phone rang. She came outside when she heard the boy cry and started to scold the dog. The next thing I saw from up the ladder, was the husband charging out of the backyard praising Dingy for saving their son's life. He proceeded to explain what happened to his wife. As I looked down, Dingy had already sauntered back to his bone in the shade and continued to gnaw on it. No big deal, just another day on the job for him. I would have to agree with the AKC's description based on my experiences with a Newfoundland. There was no need for the First Responders this time; Dingy had it under control.

At this time, I had been working at the Detroit Fire department for a little over 5 five years and was beginning to feel the daily stress from all the violence and depravity. My family had moved to Scottsdale, Arizona, almost 4 years before and my mother was wanting me to visit. I took a short vacation for a week and visited in the summer. Whoa was it hot! However, it was very safe and every day it was sunny with a bright blue sky.

"Go West Young Man" until now was a joke to me, not even a thought, but it soon became a reality. I took a leave of absence the next winter and returned to Arizona with Dingy. My folks had purchased a four, bedroom home in north Phoenix with a pool, it was nice compared to life in the big city back east. Other than Dingy digging up my mother's back yard frequently, we all got along and there was plenty of room for us.

I applied for an opportunity with the Rural Metro Fire Department in Scottsdale and was waiting to see if they would contact me. In the meantime, an old partner, Joe from the Emergency Medical Service called me and wanted me to meet him in Las Vegas. His father was a professional gambler. He bowled against and beat the Firestone Bowling Team and played tennis against Bobby Riggs (before Riggs' played Billie Jean King). He was a real character.

Well, he had a lot of gambling friends and every year they would go to Las Vegas as a group; this year the father invited Joe, his son, and he invited me. I borrowed my younger brother's purple El

Camino and headed out to Las Vegas, about 8 hours from Phoenix. I had never been to Las Vegas, and never had enough money to throw it away foolishly. I was very impressed, although the opulence made me think about all the losers that paid for it.

On the second evening Joe and I were watching one of the "Group" go on a run at the crap table. I was standing right behind him stretching my neck to try and watch. I must have gotten too close because one of the "Group's" bouncers started to move me back out of the way, but the shooter would have none of it. He said," this kid is my lucky charm." The shooter just kept winning, and soon he had over $70,000 in winnings. The next thing I knew, two bouncers, moved me out of the way and literally picked him up, one under each arm. They took him to the cashier to arrange sending most of the money back home. As they were helping him away, he glanced back at me, smiled and tossed me a black chip; I think it was worth $100.

We partied for two days with truly little sleep, not uncommon for First Responders. I got a message at around 10 PM on the second night to call home. The interview for the job with the Rural Metro Fire Department was set for the next morning at 8 AM. I was going to leave the next morning anyway, so I just moved that up and left immediately.

I arrived in Phoenix around 7 AM and had breakfast at my mother's house, several cups of coffee, a shower and drove off to the interview about 30 minutes away. I met the Fire Chief and we talked for few minutes before he gave me a written exam to complete. The time allotted was two hours, I was finished in about 45 minutes and gave him the test to grade. While I was waiting for him to grade the test, I fell asleep in the waiting room. A few minutes, later the Chief came out and woke me up. I started to explain that I was up all night and tried to apologize when he interrupted me and said, "we never had any applicant get them all correct before." Obviously, I got the opportunity, and for several months I worked as a Firefighter and First Responder in Scottsdale. The only major difficulty was the compensation was less than half of what I received in the Detroit Fire Department and eventually I returned to Detroit because of the inability to survive on what they offered in Scottsdale.

When Dingy and I returned to Detroit we rented a nice three-bedroom home with two other friends, not First Responders. I was getting a bit lonely and so I started to consciously look for a lady friend. Well, when you are looking it never works out, at least not for me. One night working the 7 PM to 7 AM shift my partner and I went into a local restaurant for a meal and I met a young waitress, named Lynn. She was a pretty, green eyed blonde, of Polish decent, but had a bad attitude. She had a rough life. Her folks were divorced, and she lived with her mother and brother in a changing violent neighborhood near the Detroit Airport. She was not a good student, and mostly just partied and never worried about tomorrow.

After a while I asked her out and she agreed to go for a ride in my Vet; I told you it was a babe magnet. We became involved over the next few months and became close, but she had some problems with drugs and her health. So, one afternoon I took her to the house where I lived. She had not slept for a couple of days. I put her upstairs in my room and placed Dingy outside the door to guard. Lynn did not know Dingy would not hurt her, all she saw was he was huge. The ploy worked, and she finally fell asleep. I tried for a couple years to get her to straighten out her life with no success; she ended up back in the same rut. It truly is a complicated world!

It is very sad to realize how poorly the United States of America, as well as most of the world's governments, have treated people with drug addiction. Addiction to drugs is different than say gambling. With drugs there are more "guns firing" in your head and body that create a psychological as well as the physical pleasure, but unfortunately also the need. The gambler only feels the "rush" when they win; obviously, Las Vegas was built on losers, so winning does not occur very often compared to the frequency of losing. The drug addict can create the "rush" anytime they can afford it and find the drugs. I am certainly not the individual that has all the answers; like most of us I do have a lot of unanswered questions.

One last thought on the extremely poor response of the world's leaders on the "war on drugs." There are thousands of lives destroyed because they were caught with cannabis, sent to prison, jobs lost, homes lost, hell even lives lost. Now, early in the 21st century there is this fantastic discovery of CBD oil that all the educated scientists and many medical professionals claim is the next greatest drug on the face of the earth to assist people with cancer, etc. Just to make sure you understand my sarcasm, they just discovered "pot", the same drug all the imprisoned folks were incarcerated for.

CHAPTER 5

On Friday and Saturday nights until early in the morning First Responders are super busy, especially in the more violent areas of the city. Responding to shootings, vehicle accidents, heart attacks, and strokes, etc., is their job. Unfortunately, like all public services some people will take advantage any way they can.

One common occurrence we experienced several times was a pregnant lady claiming she was having contractions 2 minutes apart. As explained earlier, this constitutes an emergency. We responded and carried her to the ambulance and drove to the hospital. As we were getting ready to unload the stretcher out of the ambulance, she smiled at me and proceeded to walk away. There was a grocery store that allowed food stamps across the street from the hospital. She just scammed us for a free ride to the grocery store. I caught up to her and asked her what was going on and she responded that she did not have enough money for cab fare both ways.

We also had to deal with the women who would fake passing out when their boyfriends were getting ready to go out partying without them. One incident we responded to the lady was close to 400 pounds on the third floor, with a twisting old stairway. I did the first test to see if she was faking. I will try to describe it for you. The supposed victim is laying on his/her back, you hold the arm up over the head and let go. If they are faking, the arm and hand some how falls to the floor just missing the head, if they are unconscious it will hit them in the head.

On this occasion she was good at faking, and her huge arm completely missed her head. She did not move. The next way to get a faker to respond is to take their thumb and bend it the same way it is designed to bend but apply a little more pressure. Try it yourself; most of us will stop before the excruciating pain begins. The next thing we knew was that she came off the floor, pissed off. The boyfriend got violent with us. He went down the hallway and we saw he had a shotgun; both my partner and I jumped out of the third story window landing onto the roof over the porch as the shotgun went off. Let me tell you, fear is a powerful motivator. We both rolled off the roof falling into the front bushes and ran to the ambulance and sped off. Yes, we contacted dispatch and they sent the police to arrest the boyfriend. Any police officer will tell you that "domestic violence" can escalate into the most confrontational and deadly incident.

One of the advantages of being in the first class of First Responders was having the most seniority possible. After almost 6 years of the violent neighborhoods with all the action I decide to request the Emergency Medical Service unit stationed two blocks from where I grew up on Lansdowne and Whittier. I used to walk to school right past what was only a firehouse back then; I even remember visiting my father who was stationed there in my youth.

City employees were required to live in the City of Detroit while employed by the city. Many lived on the East side of the city and back in the 60's and 70's the firefighters, police and teachers were mostly white and lived on the fringes of the city limits. These neighborhoods were very safe and peaceful compared to rest of the city and being stationed in those units was in demand. In those areas we might have 6-8 runs in a 12hour shift, in the rest of the units elsewhere in the city 15-20 runs a shift was normal, with plenty of violence and danger.

One Saturday afternoon, working in the less violent neighborhood, we responded to a vehicle accident. A juvenile escaped from jail, stole a pickup truck and tried to evade the police chasing him, getting into an accident in the process. When we got on scene the pickup was leaning up against a telephone pole all smashed up and the police had the troublemaker in handcuffs. The juvenile was about six feet tall and very muscular, had a cut over his eye from hitting the steering wheel. He was extremely drunk, and foul mouthed.

Unfortunately, I was in the jump seat, so I had to deal with this big jerk. Since he was arrested two police officers rode in the back of the ambulance with me to the hospital. Both officers were black, one male and one female. The female officer was trying to get some information out of the idiot, but he would only use racial slurs. I told him shut up and answer the officer's questions; she was being much nicer to him than I would have been. She tried again, and he spit in her face. I lost it and grabbed him by the back of the head and smashed his face into the handrail next to where he was sitting. His nose exploded all over his face. Now I was in really big trouble when we got to the hospital, as both the police officers saw me lose it!

My partner backed the ambulance up to the receiving dock and there were police officers waiting as I opened the back doors. The troublemaker immediately started screaming to the officers on the dock that I attacked him and smashed his face, which was true. So, the officer in charge asked the two black police officers, still sitting in the back of the ambulance and me what happened, I looked over at the lady officer and male officer and they were completely quiet. I sat down next to them on the bench seat and I remember we must have looked like "see no, hear no, speak no." I was extremely grateful that they lied for me. The jerk lost it and started his racial slurs again and a white police officer struck him with his night stick and threatened more if he did not shut up! Most people do not realize the bond between police officers and their partners. Each of your lives depend on each other. Skin color is not an issue, which is something the rest of the world could learn from.

On the corner of the block I grew up on, a couple of years after my parents had moved to Arizona a biker club opened a strip joint just after I was transferred to the Lansdowne and Whittier location. One evening we got a call for a lady passed out in the bathroom of the strip club. Again, I was in the jump seat. We entered the building and all these scantily dressed ladies directed me to the ladies' bathroom. I had never been in a ladies' bathroom before. In the third stall one of the dancers was passed out. She overdosed on downers, but I did not know that yet. I tried to get some answers from the dancers while I was attempting to revive her. Every time I would turn my head to talk, I would get a breast in my face because the strippers were cramming into the stall and leaning in to see how she was doing. They were concerned for their friend. Remember, I was a single, lonely, red- blooded American boy, never did I ever expect anything like this, several different sets of boobs pressed against my back. I turned my head and they were in my face. Somehow, I maintained my composure. Eventually I got one of the dancers to look in the patient's purse and we found some downers. At that point we transported her to the local hospital. I never went back to that club. Maybe I should have; however, back then I was still trying to be a good example for my partners and myself. I must admit, though, for a couple of minutes I was in lonely man's heaven!

The toll of being physically and mentally involved in so much death and violence, sickness and trauma over the years changes you. We are all a product of our environment to some degree. First Responders face the worst tragedies possible from dead babies to seniors having strokes and heart attacks. Soldiers know that they may see such trauma if they ever go to war and are on the front lines, as it is part of their job. I know many Vietnam veterans with Post Traumatic Stress Disorder, known as PTSD; these are the men that were on the front lines doing the killing or being killed themselves. It is more dangerous than most 911 calls, but not all.

The soldier is trained for war, not the First Responder. We are trained to save lives, not take them. The First Responders do not have any weapons, if you got caught with a weapon on duty you got fired. Now, this is not to say we did not hide a weapon, I had a small Derringer which I kept in my boot and never pulled it out, thank God!

The psychological affects of day in and day out being injected into these very, dangerous environments for 12 hours at a time, 7 days out of 14 adds up to about 25% of our working lives. Yes, there are vacation and other leave days, but 20% to 25% of our lives occur while we are faced with death, traumatic incidents and the mass depravity of mankind. The psychological changes we go through are not normal. Even the worst thugs only see violence occasionally, not multiple times a shift. First Responders are not originally "wired" for the danger; we are "wired" to helping those in need, not to commit violence and crimes.

Many Police Officers, Firefighters, and Emergency Medical Technicians, all First Responders, have an overwhelming percentage of marital problems due to the stressful lives they live. No one can even imagine what we see, are forced to cope with and internally evaluate as part of our jobs. This is one of those "had to be there" to understand. The stress we feel cannot be shared with our friends or spouses, especially our spouses. They innocently think we are exaggerating or over glorifying, when in reality, it is just the opposite. The blood and guts are just too painful to even discuss.

One example of that I have never told anyone, even my spouse, as it would make her cry. We responded to a 911 call that an elderly man down, no sign of any violence or trauma, so we thought it was a heart attack. As we started to remove his coat, we saw the cause of death, one small bullet wound in the chest, probably a 22 caliber. The police were chasing down the shooter and they caught him. When they searched him, they found the .22 caliber pistol and all of 25 cents in his pocket. The older gentleman had just left the post office and the bank intending to cash his social security check. However, he forgot his I.D. so he was going home to get it so he could cash his social security check. Bottom line, he was murdered for a quarter, 25 cents. What a sick world when poor seniors are stalked and killed for their pennies!

I had a hard time with that one, as well as dead newborn babies in trash cans, all these and several hundred, maybe a thousand, traumatic tragedies caused by human cruelty. It was truly a very, sick world, especially as a First Responder in the City of Detroit. Maybe in a small town or a safer city it is not as bad; however, the damage has been done to all First Responders, in some areas it is tremendously worse. At this point I started to think about moving to Arizona permanently, no more snow, no more death and depravity! Unfortunately, no job yet either.

About a month later two Emergency Medical Technicians were attacked and injured seriously, one stabbed and one beaten. I had a similar incident a few weeks later. My partner and I were responding to a call for another unit that was on a run; we pulled up in front of this tenement and I jumped out to go inside while my partner tried to park. I opened the door to this multi-family, run down- building and I was greeted by two mean Dobermans charging at me. Holy shit again! Luckily, I got out the door before they did and tried to shut it with no luck. With one Doberman at my ankles I jumped up on the parked car in front of me. My partner was coming up the street from where he parked and saw what was happening and ran back to the ambulance and backed it up towards me as I jumped! Ran! Hell, I don't know. I ran across the top of the parked cars. First the trunk, then the roof, then the hood, then the next trunk, on and on for about 8-10 cars before I got to the ambulance and jumped in when my partner, Phil, opened the passenger door while driving. It was a set-up. Apparently, another unit had responded and did not satisfy the residents, so they made a phony 911 call and set the Dobermans out to attack the EMTs when they returned. Unfortunately, we were totally unaware of what was about to happen. We contacted the police and they responded.

After evaluating my present situation, it was becoming more evident that sooner or later I would be attacked and injured because I was a white male in very, dangerous neighborhoods without any protection. The frequency of attacks started to escalate after we were on the job for 2-3 years, maybe because the public realized we did not have any weapons to protect us; I am not sure.

I decided to resign from the Fire Department. However, I did not know whether to look for work in Detroit or to move away from everything I had ever known. Leaving your home- town is not easy. In my case, I had my folks, so I decided to leave Detroit and take a chance on a new life in Arizona.

I gave notice to my roommates that I was leaving in 3 weeks, I figured they could get another roommate and I could wrap up all my loose ends like changing the name on the lease, electric and phone that were in my name along with saying goodbye to a lady friend. After three weeks I was packed, rented a little trailer to hook to my Corvette and filled it with all my junk and away I went into the next unknown step in my life.

I left on a weekday afternoon before rush hour on a dark and dreary rainy day, just what I was hoping to get away from. I got to I 40 and headed West through the wind and rain for almost 8 hours before I decided to sleep in a rest stop with a pistol in my lap, as there was no room to lay down in the Corvette. I woke up early, no problems, still windy and rainy, just nasty, so I continued driving west. The route is close to 2,000 miles and towing a trailer in bad weather took at least 40 hours of driving. However, it was no problem and I like to drive.

On the morning of the third day it was still raining and windy. I picked the wrong time to drive across the country, mid-November, nothing but rain and bad weather. I continued driving on I 40 and after several hours I thought I saw this tiny clear blue spot in the clouds off to my left, but it was so hard to see through the rain. About an hour later the rain had slowed down to a drizzle and I could clearly see this blue spot way off in the sky, to my left. I continued driving until I was too sleepy to continue and found a rest stop and went to sleep in the driver's seat for the third night in a row.

On the fourth day I was supposed to hit I-17 between Winslow and Flagstaff, Arizona where I was to turn South toward Phoenix. I was extremely excited. The rain was coming down hard and, in some stretches, there was snow. It was just a nasty day to be driving, but that blue opening in the cloudy sky was getting closer off to my left. About noon I exited I-40 freeway South to I- 17 towards Phoenix and, also directly toward that blue opening in the clouds. The closer I got to Phoenix the more prevalent the opening in the clouds. The trip from Flagstaff to Phoenix is at least 3 hours and with the rain and occasional snow it was slow moving.

Black Canyon City is the last little town before the Phoenix Metropolitan area after a long decent on I-17. As I popped out of the hilly terrain after Black Canyon City, I was suddenly looking up at a beautiful blue sky, and no more rain! The sign on the side of the road said Phoenix 18 miles and the next sign said, "Welcome to Phoenix, Valley of the Sun".

www.ingramcontent.com/pod-product-compliance
Lightning Source LLC
Chambersburg PA
CBHW071124220526
45467CB00004B/2048